AF480072

10 Minutes To Feel Less Anxious:

How To Be Proactive With Your Mental Health and Anxiety

Kyle Mitchell

Teen Social Anxiety Speaker

Dedication

I'd like to dedicate this book to my parents and everyone who has supported me over the years. I was lucky enough to grow up in a house with two parents for my entire life, which is the greatest privilege anyone can have. My parents supported me my entire childhood (and still do).

They always went out of their way to help me in any way that they could when I was struggling. When they didn't understand what I was going through, I still had them to talk to and they would always listen. With mental health not at the forefront like it is now, I am impressed by the job my parents did with me in regards to supporting me and my mental health. Not one time did they tell that it's all in my head or that I should get over it or anything like that. I can't thank them enough. This book would have never been written if my parents did not help me during the most difficult time of my life.

I love you mom and dad!

Ten Minutes to Feel Less Anxious: How to Be
Proactive with Your Mental Health and Anxiety
by Kyle Mitchell

© Copyright 2022 by Kyle Mitchell

First Edition 2022

ISBN 979-8-218-13823-3

Table of Contents

Introduction

My name is Kyle Mitchell and I struggled with social anxiety for over a decade. Now, I am a teen social anxiety & mental health international speaker & TEDx speaker with a mission to help one million teens go from socially anxious to socially confident. It took a long time to get where I am today. I can remember experiencing social anxiety as early as Kindergarten, but I did not understand what anxiety or mental health was until much later.

After overcoming my social anxiety, I thought life would be simple, but it was not. I had recently finished 4.5 years of college and graduated with a Bachelor's Degree in Marketing and Management and was eager to get a job where I could provide for my soon-to-be wife, my two-year-old, and one that was on the way. The only company willing to hire me gave me a spot as a part-time marketing intern making $10/hour. I stayed there for a while but quickly realized two things. One was that there was not an opportunity for me to move up in the company and two was that working 20 hours a week at $10/hour was not enough to provide for my family. I had to make a change.

It was one year after graduating from college when I finally swallowed my pride and took a job outside my field that paid me much better. I was working for a hospital where I talked to patients on the phone and made appointments, sent notes to their doctors, etc. To say the least, I was not thrilled with this at all. It was starting to hit me that I may have wasted four and a half years of my time preparing for something I was never going to get. I had a lot of depression and anxiety about the future of my life being something I did not want it to be. Around this time, I heard a short message from a motivational speaker named Eric Thomas who, in summary, said "you'll never get where you strive to be if you quit." I thought to myself "Wait, I can't quit! There's more I can do." This was the birth of my morning routine.

I started to become extremely invested in developing a routine filled with mental health practices that worked for me and made me feel great daily so that I could take on the challenge of not putting my degree to waste. Ninety days of doing it and applying to two different marketing jobs were all it took to get my foot in the marketing world and make enough money to provide for my family.

From that point, I was hooked and understood the power of my morning routine and began to develop it further and further to help me feel good enough to reach the goals I had for my life. It took me years of trial and error, testing, and optimizing to find the right healthy mental health morning routine for me. I authored this book with the mission of helping one million teens go from socially anxious to socially confident, as well as to express the importance of being proactive with your mental health so you can learn to live a life that is not controlled by anxiety. Enjoy!

Chapter 1: Why Do You Need a Healthy Morning Routine

I started my morning routine to begin with because I was at a point where my back was against the wall. After graduating from Indiana University Southeast with a Bachelor's degree in Marketing and Management, I was eager to start my first "real job." My wife and I just had our second child so it was perfect timing in the sense that I had the right credentials to be able to get a good-paying job and provide for my growing family.

Six months had gone by since graduation and I still had no job. I did not even have close to a real job. I was making the same money I was making straight out of high school. I could not provide for my family like I wanted to. My wife and I had to leave the house we were renting from because we could no longer afford it and my wife, two kids, and I were forced to move in with my parents. I was depressed and felt a lot of shame about this situation. I spent 4 years busting my butt to be able to create a good life for my family and I was starting to lose hope of that ever happening. I started to think that going to college was a waste of my time.

One day, I was on the way home from the YMCA with my brother listening to a Pandora station when a short motivational clip from Eric Thomas started playing. He was talking about pain. He said, "Pain is temporary but quitting lasts forever." This message in the two or three minutes he was talking spoke to my heart. It made my eyes water instantly. I thought to myself "I can't quit just because things aren't going the way I want." I needed to do something about it and keep going. This was the beginning of something that would forever change my life...I created a morning routine. I started waking up earlier and listening to him every morning on my way to my job where I took phone calls for a hospital. I did not particularly like my job and knew that it was not something I wanted to do forever so it was time to do something about it.

Every morning, I would get to my desk two hours before my shift started. I was the first one there every single morning. I got such a high from getting there first and switching the light switch on. I knew I could not control what happened, but I could control the effort I put into myself. So, that is what I did. I put work in on myself for two hours every day before work for about 3 months until I finally started to see some progress.

Right around that 3-month mark, I applied for two jobs even though I had already applied for well over one hundred jobs both in and out of state, but something told me, after a 3-month hiatus from job searching, that I should try again. To my surprise and joy, I received an email saying that they wanted to interview me. I was shocked! I had not changed anything on my resume. I didn't change the type of jobs I was applying for, but I got an interview and was one for two. That is when I realized that I did not need to change my resume to get the job. I needed to upgrade my mindset and improve my mental health to put myself in a position to be ready for a job. Doing work on myself every morning for 3 months did more than change my mindset. It made me feel happier, more optimistic, confident, and excited for opportunities to come my way. I walked into that interview with all the confidence in the world and I got it. This all happened because I started to put the effort into myself, and I showed that by performing a consistent routine. Shortly after getting this job, I started to find ways to better optimize my morning routine for my mental health. That is when I knew I could never stop doing my morning routine.

Believe it or not, you already have a morning routine whether you are conscious of it or not. It may be waking up, showering, eating, and leaving the house. I am authoring this book to teach you how you can build a HEALTHY morning routine to provide the most optimal mental health for your day and prepare your mind to manage anything the day may throw at you. There is an emphasis on "healthy" because we all have morning routines, but most people are letting life dictate their experience instead of choosing how they want to live and experience life.

By transitioning from a chaotic morning routine to a healthy one, you can make an incredible and positive impact on your life. Your happiness is based on your mental health. If your mental health is neglected, you will start to see the joy in your life decrease.

I like to think of my mental health as a battery and my morning routine as the battery charger. You wake up from a full night's rest and you have 100% battery, but the more unnecessary stimuli (information) invited into the brain and the more fast-paced decisions we make in the morning, you start to see that battery draining. This is something called decision fatigue.

Think of all the decisions you must make in the morning. Some common examples include what clothes to wear, what breakfast to eat, snoozing the alarm or not, wondering if you have enough time to [fill in the blank], stopping for coffee or making some at home, wondering if you need an umbrella or not, and the list goes on and on. Now imagine this, you wake up and you do not have those decisions to make. You follow an order of what you do every single morning without using a blip of energy from your mind. Even if this order is only 20 minutes long, that's still 20 minutes that you used efficiently and without thoughts of decision. Let me lay out an example. You wake up 20 minutes earlier, take a shower, put on the clothes you laid out the night before, drink a glass of cold water as soon as you get downstairs (because you always do that), you start making your breakfast smoothie (the same one you drink every morning), you brew your favorite coffee at home like you always do, and leave to go to work with 20 extra minutes to spare. That is just an example, but what if you did that every single morning? It would reduce the amount of stress you have in the mornings and keep that mental health battery charged as you head to work or
wherever you are going.

There have been studies done to show the impact of decision fatigue. According to a study I found in Full Focus, judges were giving parole to people in the morning much more than they did in the afternoon. Seventy percent of people seeking parole in the morning received it while only 10% of people, with simi-lar cases, seeking parole in the afternoon received it. You may be asking "Well how does that associate with mental health?"

Decision fatigue starts to turn to mental exhaustion. Another good word for it is "burnout". We have all been there and according to healthline.com, mental exhaustion can lead to depression, anxiety, cynicism, pessimism, apathy, detachment, anger, feelings of hopelessness, feeling of dread, lack of motivation, a decline in productivity, social withdrawal, and difficulty concentrating. Therefore, you need to make life easier for your brain and avoid all the unnecessary decisions in the morning. Save your battery!

We want to get rid of the things that cause decision fatigue and mental exhaustion. What happens if you start to add healthy practices and eliminate unhealthy practices for your mental health to help prepare your mind for the day ahead? That is where you can see drastic and altering life changes as I have with my morning routine. The rest of this book is all about helping you get to that life change with the optimal morning routine made for you!

Chapter 2: Common Mistakes, Misconceptions & Questions When Creating a Morning Routine

When I speak publicly, I always try to hammer in this point: you must get rid of any unhealthy habits/practices you have before adding in any healthy practices. When I first started taking my morning routine seriously, I found that I was doing things counterproductive to my mental health, which I discuss throughout this chapter.

If you are like me, you want to jump right into adding things to your routine that are going to make you feel better and prepare yourself for the day ahead. If you do that, your newly added healthy practices will only be canceled out by your "possible" long-time unhealthy habits/practices. Do not worry! By working to get rid of some of the harmful things, you will still start to feel a difference.... a potential MAJOR or even LIFE-CHANGING difference! Let me explain some common misconceptions and mistakes that I and many others have had in the beginning so you can avoid them and get right into the good stuff.

Misconception #1: YOU MUST DO THIS EVERY DAY (OR) YOU ONLY HAVE TO DO THIS ONCE A WEEK

In the beginning, I built my morning routine and was really enjoying it, but I also felt as if I could never miss a day. Of course, things happened occasionally where I did miss a day out of the week. Instead of celebrating myself for doing my morning routine six of the 7 days of the week, I focused on the 1 day I missed because I thought I had to be perfect. By doing this, I would spiral downwards and feel bad about myself when I should have been proud of myself for doing it most of the week. Do not make the same mistake I made. Give yourself realistic expectations.

On the other side of the spectrum, is the thought that you can do this once a week and it will create amazing results for you. It will not. Having a daily morning routine is training your brain for less anxiety and increased happiness and doing it once a week is not enough to train it.

The key thing to note here is that consistency is important. I love the way Sashin Govender said it on my podcast, The Social Ninjas. "Consistency is currency." What does that mean though? I take it to mean that what you are striving for is defined by your consistent actions to achieve it.

It is important to remember that consistency is different from perfection. If you treat the challenge of building a morning routine as something you must do perfectly, you are going to disappoint yourself. Perfection with your morning routine is not possible so do not hold yourself to those standards. This is something I had to learn the hard way.

You may be asking yourself "how many times a week do I need to do a morning routine?" I will talk about that in a later chapter. For now, we are just focusing on misconceptions and mistakes.

Misconception #2: THERE IS A ONE-SIZE FITS ALL ROUTINE (AKA THE PERFECT ROUTINE)

Everyone is different therefore everyone's process is different. You have probably heard this about diets, exercise, etc. You must find what works for you. There is a reason why I am not telling you to do exactly what I do every morning. What works for me very well may not work for you and what works for you may not work for me. Morning routines are going to look different for everyone depending on many factors like: if you have kids, you work the night shift, you live with four roommates, you have a different personality type than me, and/or your brain is wired much different than mine. That is why when I start talking about creating your routine later in this book, I am very adamant about evaluating your routine to see what works great and what doesn't. As I said, I will get more into testing and how to do that
properly later in this book.

Misconception #3: YOU HAVE TO CUT YOUR SLEEP DOWN TO HAVE A GOOD ROUTINE

I believed this at the beginning of my routine-building journey. I believed that if I got 8 hours of sleep, I was being lazy and that I could do better. This is not true. When I was trying to run off 4 to 5 hours of sleep each night, my mental health deteriorated. I was much more anxious and impatient, and it became something that wasn't fun anymore. I could do it for 2 days in a row but after that, I went downhill. That was something I evaluated and optimized for myself. I altered the time I was going to bed and waking up. After doing that, I was feeling much better. Find the proper amount of sleep that works for YOU.

I found that if I get 6 hours of sleep each night, I run like a well-oiled machine. I also found out that this also depends on my current life situation. As I am authoring this book, I have a lot more on my plate than what I was doing a year ago. Trying to go on 6 hours of sleep was not cutting it anymore so I bumped it up to 8 hours. It took me much longer than I would like to admit to accepting the fact that I needed that extra 2 hours, but that is what I need (at least right now). What do you need?

Misconception #4: "I'M NOT A MORNING PERSON"

I have a whole section dedicated to this misconception because while I have not personally struggled with this mindset...MANY do. That is what it is. It is a mindset. You're not a morning person because you are constantly telling yourself that you are not. You are someone who believes this about yourself. Know that you can be a "morning person" and I will show you how later.

Now it is time for some of the most common mistakes that I have made, and many others have, when starting a morning routine.

Mistake #1: GOING FROM NO MORNING ROUTINE TO A COMPLEX ONE

Start slow. The last thing you want to do is set yourself up for failure by trying to stick to a complex routine that is almost impossible to stay consistent with. When you are not staying consistent, missing multiple days, and not having time to get through all the practices, you can start to feel bad about yourself, which is counterproductive to what you are trying to achieve.

Plus, if you try to start with a morning routine with a variety of practices, it is impossible to tell what works well for you and what does not. Testing becomes impossible. I will cover how to start creating your morning routine slowly later.

Mistake #2: NOT GIVING A PRACTICE PROPER TESTING TIME

You know now that you should be testing out different practices because of what we talked about earlier. There is no one-size-fits-all. That is why you must evaluate to see what works for you. The big mistake here is not giving a practice enough testing time to determine if it is helpful or not. So how long should you evaluate a practice in your routine?

I would say at least a month. You might find out much sooner than that if something works or is terrible for you, but a month should give you a good look to see if something is good for you or not. To help with testing, you can use a journal to write down how you feel after your morning routine and how you feel when going to bed. This way you are not left wondering at the end of the month whether that was something valuable to you or not.

Remember, some of the practices you will try will take time to see/feel results. The most common example I hear is: "I tried meditation, but it didn't work for me." When I hear this, I usually ask how long they have been doing it. Most of the time, the person will reply that they tried it a couple of times. Trying anything a couple of times is going to be hard to gauge what result it will provide you. Be patient. This is not a race. This is a marathon and building a great morning routine for you will be worth it.

Mistake #3: BUILDING TOO QUICKLY

This goes back to the point that this is a marathon, not a sprint. Trying to add too many practices to your routine at once has many disadvantages.

The first disadvantage goes back to testing. If you are adding two or more practices for your mental health at the same time, how are you supposed to know which ones are working or not working? You cannot. I know it is time-consuming to have to add one at a time, but that is the only way to do it and have a morning routine that works great for you.

The second disadvantage is a piggyback off the first mistake I mentioned of going from zero to many too quickly. You do not want to overwhelm yourself and cause inconsistency with your routine. Do not make this mistake. It will waste your time and prolong your finding a great morning routine.

Now, let us spend some time over the most frequent questions I hear when creating and starting a morning routine.

Question #1: How long should my morning routine be?

This goes back to how everyone is different and there is no one size fits all routine. In the early days of my morning routine journey, I built and maintained a routine that took me over 2 hours to complete and I have also performed routines that took 10 minutes. I suggest you keep it short, at least to start with, and build it out as you like if you can stay consistent with it. The key thing to remember here is the length of your morning routine does not determine the quality of your routine. Your morning routine is not going to automatically fill you with more benefits for your mental health because you added 30 minutes to it. A five or 10-minute routine can be just as powerful as one that is 30 minutes long.

Question #2: Is it okay to take a break from your routine?

Yes, it is okay to take a break. It all depends on what you need. For example, my mother-in-law passed away in March of 2020 and it was an especially tough time for my wife. I stopped my morning routine for a while so I could stay up with her and be there with her and not have to worry about waking up before the kids did so I could do my routine. I had a moment of shame when this happened, but do not let that consume you. You should not feel ashamed of pausing your morning routine when you need to.

There are also times when you shouldn't take a break, but you feel like you should. It is a complex feeling wondering if you should take a break from your routine because of anxiety or depression knowing that a morning routine can help with those things. You can take a break if you need to, but do not go more than a few days as you may lose your consistency and find yourself going down a slippery slope with your mental health. Take a few days off and get back on the horse knowing that what you are going to do is going to make you feel better.

Question #3: Should I continue my morning routine when I go on vacation or go out of town?

I put this question in because this was a question I had for myself for a long time. Here is what I produced after many vacation morning routine trials and errors. If your morning routine is short around 10 to 15 minutes, you should do it while out of town. There is no reason you shouldn't. It is not worth throwing yourself completely off and having to try to get back in the swing of things when you get back. Plus, you want to feel good on vacation too, right?

If you have a longer morning routine, it is a different story. This is the scenario I specifically struggled with. I had an exceptionally long (2+hour) morning routine but could not commit to it while on vacation. I wanted to allow myself to relax, stay up late, sleep in, and do all that good stuff you do on vacation. My problem was that I would not do a routine at all and after being on vacation for a week, I would spend close to a month trying to get back where I left off. I produced a new strategy for my morning routine this past vacation I took. I created a shortened version of my routine that only lasted 10 minutes. This way I was still taking care of my mental health but also able to enjoy my vacation and relax. When I got back home, I was able to easily transition back into my normal morning routine.

Question #4: Where do I start?

I have dedicated the entire next chapter to answering that question.

Chapter 3: HOW TO GET STARTED

Getting yourself to start doing your morning routine is the hardest part, which is why this chapter is so crucial! Once you start feeling your anxiety decrease, stress decrease,

happiness increase, self-worth increase, mood increase, and your overall mental health increase, it is easy to keep doing it. You started doing something that makes you feel great so why would you stop? You would not. That is why having a strong "why" for your morning routine is necessary for getting yourself started with a healthy and consistent morning routine.

Developing a Strong "Why"

What I mean by this is developing the reason you are doing this. One of the biggest reasons people (including myself in the past) quit on a goal is because their "why" is...to be frank...garbage. Think of the common example of wanting to lose weight. If you ask someone who has a goal to lose 50 pounds and you ask them "Why?" you will most often hear answers like these: "I want to look better.", "I want to impress my crush.", "I want to look good in my wedding dress.", "I want to look good on the beach this summer.", etc. Now let's compare those "why's" to some strong "why's" like "I want to feel better so I can be a better parent to my children.", "I want to be able to see my grandkids born.", "I want to improve my health so I can be sure to be around for the long haul for my kids and not leave them with a single parent." Now, if you were betting on someone who you thought would lose the fifty pounds solely based on their "why", who would you choose? The person who wants to look good in their swimsuit or the person who wants to lose weight because they don't want their kids to lose a parent at such an early age. The answer is the latter. The reason is because that person's why is outside themselves. They are not doing it for selfish reasons. They are doing it for someone they love. Make your "why" about something or someone other than yourself.

"I'm Not a Morning Person"

The most common excuse I hear for not doing a morning routine is "I'm not a morning person." I say excuse because that is what it is. It is not like you're missing the morning person gene. Your thoughts around mornings might be negative. You might casually say to your friends frequently "I'm not a morning person." or "I'm a night owl." And you would be right because what you say to yourself is what you become. So, if you've been telling yourself that you are not a morning person, you have spent years training your brain to think and believe that you are indeed not a morning person. Though you spent years of training (unintentionally), you can retrain your brain within a month or even days. Before I tell you how, I want to share an impressive story of someone who went from not being a morning person to waking up nine million people every morning.

That man would be Steve Harvey. Steve is most notably known for his talk shows, being the host of the Family Feud, and being a comedian, but he did not start there. He talks about

a time when he had no job, had no money, and just started
selling stuff with Amway. His Amway trainer/mentor started to
call him at about 5:30 AM with excitement in his voice saying,
"Hey, Steve! It is good to be alive! Today is going to be a great
day! Everything good with you?" Steve replied, "Yeah, man.
I'm just asleep." His trainer hung up. His trainer called him
again the next morning saying the same thing. His trainer
did this for about 3 weeks until he asked Steve, "Why do you
answer the phone like that? What is wrong with you? If you
are not going to show people that you are happy to be alive
this morning, you should at least let God know." The next
morning Steve was up at 4:30 AM waiting on the edge of his
bed for his trainer to call. He did and Steve excitedly answered
"Hey John! What's up, man? Today is going to be a great day!
I'm so happy to be up this morning!" His trainer replied, "That
sounds about right." From that point forward, Steve decided to approach mornings with gratitude and stopped telling
himself that he was not a morning person. Shortly thereafter,
he was offered two million dollars to host a radio program
in Chicago where he was the person who helped over nine
million people wake up every single morning. The moral of the
story is that being a "morning person" is a choice. Choose to
make it. Here's how you can do it.

First, you may have to alter your sleeping schedule for you
to get up in the morning and feel great. If you regularly go to
bed at 1 AM and now you are trying to get up at 5 AM, that is
going to be terrible. When I first decided to make a morning
routine, I knew I had to get up earlier. I started by getting up
30 minutes earlier than usual, which meant me waking up at
6 AM. In turn, I went to bed 30 minutes earlier. I did not stop

there. My goal was to be able to wake up at 3 AM and feel great mentally and not feel like I was dying. Every two weeks, I would go to bed 15 minutes earlier and wake up 15 minutes earlier. So, after waking up at 6 AM for 2 weeks, I started waking up at 5:45 AM and going to bed 15 minutes earlier. This process worked very well for me, and I eventually got down to waking up at 3 AM every morning without feeling like I was going to pass out. This process allows your body to slowly transition and change your body's internal clock without completely messing you up. Can you imagine trying to go from waking up at 6:30 AM to 3 AM in one day?

Second, change your thoughts around mornings. Train your brain to think of mornings differently. One of the most effective and efficient ways of doing this is called "mirror work." Mirror work is standing in the mirror, looking at your-self in the mirror, and stating "I am" statements to yourself that you want to believe. This is part of my morning routine, but you can do this any time of day or night. Saying things like "I am someone who enjoys the morning.", "I am a morning person.", "I love mornings", "I feel happiest in the mornings!", etc. are all great affirmations to use to retrain your subcon-scious mind to enjoy mornings. There is one last crucial step you must take to make this work.

You must believe what you are saying. You must give energy to what you are saying. You cannot speak blandly to the mirror while thinking about how "stupid this is." Trust me, this will feel stupid the first few times. To create the belief (that you do not currently believe), play the music that raises your body's frequency and energy. When I say play, I mean BLARE it! Find a song to play in the background that really gets you going while you are doing the mirror work. I use a playlist on Spotify that I found called "Motivational Soundtrack Music." and it is amazing! Playing the music in the background while you are talking to yourself in the mirror will help you believe what you are saying and in turn, will train your subconscious mind to not want or hope but to believe!

Lastly, your morning routine is meant to be enjoyable. This should not be something you dread. Something you can do to make it more of a ritual that you love is to use the scents of candles or oil diffusers to lift your mood. This is something I like to do off and on. When I go downstairs to meditate, I like to light a candle. It helps me get a little bit more enjoyment out of what I am doing. I make it special because I won't light that candle unless I am starting my routine, so my brain associates that good smell I love with the morning. Do these three things and you can "trick" your brain into loving mornings.

Make Room for the Good

Before you start creating a routine and adding healthy practices, you need to take an assessment of your typical morning as it is now. You need to make sure you are not enrolled in any habits that are detrimental to your morning routine. This is important because adding healthy practices to your routine while you are performing negative habits causes them to cancel out. You want to feel good after doing your morning routine, not neutral. Let's make sure you are not doing any of the following habits that are negative to your mental health.

Before reading on, remember that it is okay if you find yourself doing some of these or all of them. That is just more opportunity to grow the strength of your mental health! So, if you are doing all of these, be excited for the life change you are about to have. If you are doing none of these, be grateful that you can get right to adding a practice to your morning routine.

First, never hit snooze on your alarm or set multiple alarms. According to PsychologyToday, this activates the fight or flight function of your brain, and it has been shown that it causes anxiety. The last thing you want is to start your morning feeling anxious. An even better way to wake up is to do so without any alarm. The alarm itself can trigger that fight or flight. This is something I still work on. You will notice that once you have trained your body clock to go to bed and wake up at the same time every day, you will start to wake up naturally minutes before your alarm goes off. I can get up without an alarm sometimes, but I always set it just in case I don't for whatever reason.

Next, remove the clutter. You want the area you are going to be spending your time during your morning routine to be clean and clutter-free. You want an environment that evokes peace and happiness. When your area is dirty and cluttered it can make you feel that way as well even if you do not realize it. Trust me, you will realize the difference between cluttered to clean when walking into the room to perform your morning routine.

I perform my morning routine in my living room. It is very spacious and peaceful there, but I also have three kids, so they spend a lot of time there during the day and night. They can create quite a mess. I try to make sure that the room is nice and tidy before we go to bed so I do not walk into my dark living room, get upset because I stepped on a barbie, and then flip the light switch on to realize that the place is a mess. I am speaking from experience when I say that it impacts the start of my day and my mental health. I want to start my day feeling good and peaceful and if I walk into a room like that, that is not what I feel.

This next one is the one that gives people the most trouble. It's extremely hard because most of us are addicted to it.... our phones! My rule is to not use the phone for the first hour I am awake. The reason is that it is information overload way too early for your brain. According to Business 2 Community, over 80% of people look at their phones before they brush their teeth, which means many of us are looking at our phones as soon as we wake up and before we even get out of bed. Imagine going from your most peaceful and relaxed state of mind (sleep) to checking your email or Facebook with tons of incoming stimuli for your brain. It throws your brain way out of whack, and I can speak from experience.

When I was in college, I would check my phone first as soon as I woke up. I would end up spending 20+ minutes laying in my bed and scrolling through my newsfeed. Not only was it a waste of time, but it made me feel "blah" the rest of the day. After feeling like that for so long, I decided to delete the Facebook app from my phone so I would not be tempted to look at it when I woke up. I started to feel a massive shift in my mental health and the energy I felt throughout the day. I no longer felt like I was living in a fog because I was living more in

the present. Even after sharing that story, many
people are often still hesitant to give up their favorite drug,
the phone. Maybe you are thinking the same. Take this
challenge and you will be able to feel an enormous difference.
Go 1 week without looking at your phone for the first hour of
the day. That's all it takes, and I guarantee you will feel better
than you did before.

Officially Getting Started

Now, we are moving on to what you have been waiting for. I
am going to show you how to start creating and implementing
your morning routine. First, I want you to go grab a piece of
paper or open the notes on your phone. You will use this to
create your schedule for your morning routine. This will begin
noticeably short as we will only start with one practice. Write
down what time you are going to wake up. Next, write down
what time you will start your first practice. You may want to
give yourself a few minutes to use the bathroom, get a drink,
etc. It may look something like this:

6:00 AM - Wake up
6:05-6:15 - Meditate (or whatever you choose)

You are probably wondering what your first practice should be
and what options you have. Do not worry! We are discussing a
wide variety of mental health practices that you can include in
your morning routine in the next chapter.

Chapter 4: The Top Mental Health Practices to Choose From for Your Morning Routine

There is no one-size-fits-all for which practices to include in your morning routine, and that is why I produced nine of the absolute best practices you can include in your morning routine. Remember, we are all different. Starting all nine of these is not going to undoubtedly give you the ultimate morning routine and mental health. These might work great for you but there may be some that do not so keep that in mind and always TEST! My gentle suggestion for everyone is to start with this one mental health practice: Meditation!

Dr. Joseph Annabali defines mindfulness (meditation) as "a way of being–a way of looking inside oneself, of being aware of awareness, of paying attention nonjudgmentally to the unfolding of experience." Therefore, I believe that it is the ultimate tool at your disposal if you struggle with any kind of anxiety like I have. I wanted to have data on meditation because I was not fully bought into it. I found it when I started reading Dr. Annabali's book, Reclaim Your Brain: How to Calm Your Thoughts, Heal Your Mind, and Bring Your Life Back Under Control where he says "Meditation helps to eliminate feelings of anxiety and anger. Using MRI scans, researchers at the University of Wisconsin looked at the brains of meditators and discovered that during meditation their amygdala (the part of the brain responsible for the fight-or-flight impulse) switches off, and the prefrontal cortex (the area of the brain responsible for feelings of peace, compassion, and happiness) lights up." Annabali (p. 62) There are hundreds of studies that have been done on meditation and mental health/anxiety. The truth is that meditation is one of the single greatest tools for anxiety and general mental health, but meditation can also be a daunting tool for many, including myself in the past. Dr. Annabali's book, Reclaim Your Brain: How to Calm Your Thoughts, Heal Your Mind, and Bring Your Life Back Under Control

I first tried meditation in college. My brother told me about it. I did no research. I grabbed my phone, set a timer for 10 minutes, and sat in the dark of my room with my eyes closed. The entire time I was meditating I was thinking about how much time was left. "It's probably about 5 minutes left." I would think. "Surely it has been 10 minutes." It felt like such a waste of time, so I quit doing it for a few years.

After my continued learning of mental health and anxiety, I stumbled upon guided meditations, specifically from an app called Headspace. With guided meditations, I was able to listen to directions which were extremely helpful since I was a complete meditation newbie and had no idea what I was do-ing. The guided meditation worked extremely well for me and after a couple of months, I started to see/feel some amazing results. I became much less reactionary to things that came up in my life and the biggest benefit was it gave me such a strong awareness of my thoughts. My thoughts stopped running in the background of my subconscious. Now, I was able to pinpoint a thought and how it made me feel, which gave me the ability to dig deeper into the connection between my thoughts and how I felt. As I have continued further in my education about meditation, I have learned and felt some extremely wild and amazing benefits.

About a year ago, I started meditating using some of Dr. Joe Dispenza's guided meditations and I could not believe what happened. His meditation routines are long compared to most. The guided meditation I want to tell you a story about is about 45 minutes. This meditation is designed to take you through the eight energy centers of your body and cleanse you of toxins and bring your energy to the top energy center. After doing this meditation for a few days, I noticed that my stomach started to feel sick at the same time during the meditation every day. When I say I felt sick, I mean that my stomach just felt kind of nasty. I knew this couldn't be a coincidence, so I started to research on Google why this was happening and what I found out blew my mind. That feeling I was having was my body getting rid of the toxins I had in my body. I even read that when people go to Dr. Joe Dispenza's retreats, many will have flu-like symptoms for about a week afterward because of the mind/body transformation happening. I tell you this story because your mind controls how you feel, and you can train your mind with meditation. Therefore, I believe meditation is a wonderful place to start your morning routine. Five to 10 minutes in the morning is all you need.

Before I move on to the next practice you could add to your morning routine, I want to advise that you do not go straight to doing long meditations like Dr. Joe Dispenza's. Remember, you want to start slow and if you have never meditated before and you jump straight to doing it for 45 minutes, you will burn out.

This next practice is simple and so powerful, which is why I love it! Make your bed after you get up. It is a wonderful way to get a win for your day first thing in the morning. It makes me feel great and accomplished, plus it makes my room much more presentable and less stimulating to my mind when I come back to it to go to sleep later that night. According to Best Mattress Brand, they surveyed 500 people who make their bed and 500 who do not, 74% of people who make their bed have a feeling of accomplishment at the end of the day while only 50% of non-bed-makers. What is great is that this only takes a few minutes so literally anyone can do it. My kids have been making their bed since they were 4 years old so you can too!

Many (including myself) have used visualization to overcome fear and anxiety about specific situations, events, and more. It is also used to help visualize your future self and what you want that to look like. You may have heard things like "You can't be it until you believe it." This is how you can cultivate that belief, even if it seems so far away or impossible.

I do a lot of speaking on the topic of mental health and my story with social anxiety and general anxiety. This was (and sometimes still is) nerve-wracking to me. I like to visualize daily up to a month before doing a speech. For example, I got a speaking gig at a middle school where I was going to be speaking to over 600 students. I had never spoken to an audience of this size, so I used visualization to train my brain to be ready for it. I would lay on the couch every morning and spend time going through the entire process of me speaking. I would visualize myself walking into the building (I Googled it, so I knew what it looked like). I visualized walking onto the stage in front of 600 students. I visualized them smiling and laughing as I was speaking. I visualized them engaged. I visualized myself feeling completely confident and comfortable while I was speaking. After doing that for a month, I had all the confidence in the world while giving my speech about mental health. I felt so much more comfortable than I thought I would have been, and it is all because I visualized my whole experience. This is also a very great technique for people with a fear of flying, job interviews, negotiations, and so much more!

I hated reading growing up. I did everything possible to not read. I went through 4 years of college without reading. Today, I love reading! I love reading books about personal development. This was something I added to my routine in the early days of creating my routine and I have never taken it out. When I am reading (learning) I feel so good about myself. It boosts the self-esteem and confidence that I have in myself. I have talked with many others about this and that's why they read too. It is a fantastic way to keep your brain active and to keep growing as an individual. If you are not learning, you are dying.

In my living room, I have a giant sign that reads "Attitude of Gratitude Open 7 Days a Week | 365 Days a Year." Gratitude is such an important part of not only my morning routine but my life. According to Tremendousness's YouTube video "Science of Gratitude", research shows that an attitude of gratitude can measurably improve your overall well-being. It has also been proven to improve mental health, improve physical health, boost your self-esteem, enhance your sleep,

and increase your empathy. What's even cooler is that regular gratitude practice will train your brain to appreciate and retain positive thoughts and block out negative ones.
https://youtu.be/JMd1CcGZYwU

This is one we should all include in our morning routine as we start to build. It has too many benefits and is too simple not to. Here is how I practice every morning. I open my small notebook (gratitude journal) on my desk, and I write five things that I am grateful for in the past 24 hours. Staying with the past 24 hours keeps your gratitude from getting stale and writing the same things repeatedly. Another fun way to practice gratitude is to write thank you notes to people. You do not have to send them. Writing them by itself gives you the benefits of gratitude but sending them to
people is also an amazing gesture.

If you are looking to cultivate belief in yourself, in your dreams, or change your mindset, self-affirmations are the key. Self-affirmations are statements that you create for yourself that start with "I am…". With these statements, you can retrain your subconscious mind to believe these state-ments. It is almost like tricking your brain, but not really. For example, the common one that people use, including myself, is "I am confident." Confidence is not tangible. Confidence is purely a belief and a mindset that one has. By repeating this statement to yourself and training your brain, you will start to believe you are confident, therefore, you are confident. Like everything, there is a right way and a wrong way to do this.

You cannot just simply utter out some statements and think

that is going to retrain your brain. You have to say it as if you already believe it...even if you do not. You must say it with emotion. Next, you need to say these statements to yourself in the mirror. You are talking to yourself, so you need to see yourself. There is much more power when these are done looking at yourself in the mirror. The last piece to complete this powerful self-affirmation practice is to play music while doing this. You need to play the music that hypes you up and makes you feel motivated. This creates energy in your body and raises your body's frequency. This also makes the emotion/belief of these statements to yourself start to come out more naturally. This is something I do every morning and my favorite part of the morning just because after I finish with those, I am mentally ready to take on anything the day brings.

Here is a list of some examples of self-affirmations you can use.

I am amazing!
I am unstoppable!
I love myself!
I am happy!
I am confident!
I have value!
I am loved!
I am carefree!
I am brave!
I live in this moment!

Of course, these are just suggestions. Create them based on what you are needing in your life.

If you would like to know more about the science behind self-affirmations and why and how they work, check out Dr. Joe Dispenza's TED Talk called "How to Rewire Your Brain." https://youtu.be/ZjNSwUb_Sj4

"Inspiration fires you up; motivation keeps you burning."
- Stuart Aken

I love including something to motivate myself in my morning routine. For me, this is usually watching a motivational YouTube video, which there is no short supply of. I watch one short video as the last thing I do in my routine, so I move on to the rest of my day motivated to take it on. To me, it completes the morning routine experience.

Here are some of my favorite motivational YouTube channels:

Dr. Billy Alsbrooks https://www.youtube.com/c/BillyAlsbrooks

Etthehiphoppreacher https://www.youtube.com/c/etthehiphoppreacher

Evan Carmichael https://www.youtube.com/c/Evancarmichael

HESMotivation https://www.youtube.com/c/HESMotivationOfficial

Motiversity https://www.youtube.com/c/motiversity

MulliganBrothers https://www.youtube.com/user/mulliganbrother

The Official Steve Harvey https://www.youtube.com/channel/UCNnnebGh-mlJ8MQ4X1HwphRw

Walter Bond https://www.youtube.com/c/WalterBond

There are tons of motivational content out there. Do some research and see what really resonates with you.

According to the Mayo Clinic, exercising for 30 minutes a day for three days a week reduces anxiety, depression, and social withdrawal. It also improves cognitive function and self-esteem. What is great is you don't have to be lifting weights or doing sprints. A simple brisk walk for 30 minutes has the same impact as running or lifting weights for 30 minutes.

If exercise has never really been your thing, here is what I do to keep myself going. Make it fun! Exercising should not be a dreadful practice. For example, I do not like running. It is boring to me. I like to lift weights though. To me, that is fun. On days that I do want to get some cardio in, I will go play basketball instead. Making exercise fun is vital to staying consistent with doing it.

They are not lying when they say breakfast is the most important meal of the day. According to pubmed.gov, "those who consumed...breakfast each day were less depressed, less emotionally distressed, and had lower levels of perceived stress than those who did not eat breakfast each day." Breakfast should be a part of everyone's morning routine for better mental health. Do not skip breakfast! I repeat... DO NOT SKIP BREAKFAST! https://pubmed.ncbi.nlm.nih. gov/10367010/

Now that I got the message that you should eat breakfast, here is a way to make your breakfast even more powerful by using intermittent fasting. Intermittent fasting is different for everyone and primarily means that you are fasting intermittently. Some people may fast for two days or some fast for 8 hours every day. I fast for about the first five and a half to 6 hours of being awake each day until I eat. "According to the Journal of Nutrition Health & Aging, after 3 months of intermittent fasting, study participants improved moods and decreased tension, anger, and confusion." Another study also showed that it had "significant improvements in emotional well-being and depression."

Chapter 5: Plan B: When S!*& Hits the Fan

One of the first big struggles I had with my morning routine was contemplating whether I should use it when my environment had changed. For example, going out of town, going on vacation, etc. What I ended up doing was skipping my morning routine when I was not in my normal environment with my rationale being that this should be a time to relax. Doing this, made getting back on my morning routine when I would get back extremely hard! I would be starting from square one where I would have to work my way up to rebuilding my routine. It would take me upwards of a month to get back on track. It was not working out at all for me.

I eventually met in the middle between doing my full morning routine and doing nothing at all because I was on vacation. I created what I call my "Plan B" morning routine to use anytime I am outside my normal environment. If one of my kids keeps me up late last night because they are sick, I am not going to be able to get up as early in the morning as I usually do. In the past, I would let this drag me down and beat myself up for not being able to do my routine. Not anymore! Now, I do my quick "Plan B" morning routine and I am good to go for the day!

At the beginning of creating your morning routine, you should not need a "Plan B" morning routine because your routine should only be one thing and you cannot shorten it. This is something to keep in mind as you continue to build out your routine because there will come a time when "x" happens out of nowhere and you are left scrambling. Do not scramble. Use your "Plan B".

Getting Back on Track When (Not IF) You Fall Off

I do not mean to sound negative. I want to give you realistic expectations. Things will happen and you will fall off your routine. You might get the flu, a family member may pass, you may not be able to sleep for several days in a row, your kids may wake up during your morning routine time, etc. All these are things that can throw you off your morning routine...and that is OKAY! This is life. Do not go into this thinking that you will never miss a day or ever fall off the wagon. You will. So, let's prepare for when that happens and how to get back at it.

First, be kind to yourself about falling off. Tell yourself that you are doing your best. In the early days, I would fall off my morning routine occasionally for various things. When my wife and I had my son, he would go through periods where he would keep us up at night and/or wake up at the same time I had my alarm set. I was extremely negative and disappointed in myself for not being able to keep my morning routine going during this time. Why? It was not my fault for not being able to do my morning routine. I acted this way towards myself because I had a vision of perfection with my morning routine. I had no room for error in my routine. Be kind to yourself be-cause things are going to happen.

Second, take the time you need and get back on track when it is possible. That is all you can ultimately do. Sometimes, depending on the situation, you can improvise and still do your Plan B morning routine. When my son was first born, he would wake up many times as I was about to go downstairs to meditate. I got tired of not being able to at least meditate so I took him with me. He would sit on my lap in the pitch-black living room as I meditated in a soothing guided meditation. Unbelievably, he sat there with me very content. He even fell asleep sometimes! Like I said, improvising isn't always an option, but it can be extremely helpful. In the end, you need to decide what you need to do based on your situation. My best piece of advice is to give yourself some grace and take that break if trying to fit in the morning routine is nearly impossible. Just get back at it as soon as possible. Try not to go longer than a week or two if you can help it.

In summary, things are going to happen. Make sure you are prepared for it with a Plan B morning routine. When Plan B does not work and you fall off, give yourself grace and get back on as soon as possible.

Chapter 6: Evening Routines Help Your Morning Routine

This book is about morning routines, but I want to talk a little bit about an evening routine. An evening routine is beneficial for many reasons, like better sleep, less stress going to bed, and feelings of relaxation, but the benefit I want to focus on is how it helps your morning routine. Here are a few things you can do to decrease your decision fatigue in the morning and increase the efficiency of your morning routine.

Set your clothes out the night before. This simple act has such a powerful impact. Remember, EVERY decision you make increases your mental fatigue. Why would you waste your brain's energy on deciding what to wear that day when you can make that decision before you go to bed? If you are like me and go to the gym in the morning, pack your gym bag the night before. This is a huge energy saver for me as I do not have to worry about getting a bag, packing extra clothes, grabbing deodorant, having a towel, and my extra set of shoes that are not my gym shoes. Another side benefit is that this saves you time in the morning.

Write down your goals for tomorrow. This way you are not spending time and your BRAIN'S ENERGY trying to think of what you want to do that day. Use the energy you have left over the night before to do this. When you are doing this, do not try to write a list of twenty things you want to do. We do not want to set ourselves up for failure. I would try and limit yourself to three things you can accomplish tomorrow. That number is not overwhelming and completely doable. To piggyback on this, you should also write down three things that you accomplished today...big or small. These could be the three goals you had set out for the day, or they could just be things you are proud to have accomplished this day. This is an effective way to close the loop on your day and end the day feeling good about what you have done.

Another one that I like to do at night that I also do in the morning is self-affirmations. When I was growing up living in my parent's house, my mom would always tell me to read over my study material for the test the next day right before I went to bed. She said this helps as this is the last thing that will be in your brain as you go to sleep. It is almost like your brain does some studying for you while you are sleeping. And it works! Every time I did this, I retained the information a little bit better than times that I did not do this. This process also works for self-affirmations. While you are asleep, your brain is bouncing around the self-affirmations like "I am confident.", "I am amazing.", "I love myself." which is getting some good brain training in. For me, I wake up a little bit easier when I do these at night and have a less tough time trying to get my mind in the right space when I awaken.

Do not let this evening routine suggestion overwhelm you. If this is too much now, skip it. Focus on the morning routine. Once you have the morning routine built out and rocking and rolling then you can add this in to enhance your morning routine even further, but please do not try to do this all at once.

CONCLUSION

You have obtained a great deal of valuable information that will be transformative to your life. We talked about how to be proactive with your mental health and anxiety by developing a custom-fit morning routine for YOU! Not only that but we went through many challenges you may come across along the way.

Thank you for being an important part of the mission of helping one million teens go from socially anxious to socially confident. To help reach the one million, I need you to not only act on the practices of this book but to also share with those around you your struggles, your process, your results, and the information that you learned while reading this book.

Confidence is contagious, and if we can build it for ourselves, we can build it for others.

For more tools and resources to help improve your mental health, you can go to my website, www.socialanxietykyle. com, where you can find my TEDx talk, free resources like my "3 Steps to Take Back Control From Social Anxiety", and my social media channels to connect with me.

Bibliography

Amen, Clinic. "7 Incredible Things Intermittent Fasting Does for Your Brain." Amen Clinics 7 Incredible Things Intermittent Fasting Does for Your Brain Comments, https://www.amenclinics.com/blog/7-incredible-things-intermittent-fasting-does-for-your-brain/#:~:text=Research%20in%20the%20Journal%20of,tension%2C%20anger%2C%20and%20confusion.

Annibali, Joseph A, and Joseph A A Annibali. "Becoming Mindful." Reclaim Your Brain: How to Calm Your Thoughts, Heal Your Mind, and Bring Your Life Back under Control, Avery Publishing, 2015, pp. 62–62.

Mayo Clinic, Staff. "Depression and Anxiety: Exercise Eases Symptoms." Mayo Clinic, Mayo Foundation for Medical Education and Research, 27 Sept. 2017, https://www.mayoclinic.org/diseases-conditions/depression/in-depth/depression-and-exercise/art-20046495.

Monroy, Lauren. "Can Making the Bed in the Morning Make You Happier?" Best Mattress Brand, 13 Aug. 2022, https://bestmattress-brand.org/making-the-bed/.

Pelusi, Nando. "I Can't Stand That Noise." Psychology Today, Sussex Publishers, https://www.psychologytoday.com/au/articles/200804/i-cant-stand-noise.

Santos-Longhurst, Adrienne. "Mental Exhaustion: Definition, Causes, Symptoms, and Treatment." Healthline, Healthline Media, 31 Mar. 2022, https://www.healthline.com/health/mental-exhaustion#symptoms.

Smith, A P. "Breakfast and Mental Health." International Journal of Food Sciences and Nutrition, U.S. National Library of Medicine, https://pubmed.ncbi.nlm.nih.gov/10367010/.
Spillane, James. "80% Of Smartphone Users Check Their Phones Before Brushing Their Teeth ... And Other Hot Topics." Business 2 Community, 5 Apr. 2013, https://www.business-2community.com/social-media-articles/80-of-smartphone-users-check-their-phones-before-brushing-their-teeth-and-other-hot-topics-0457524.

Tremendousness, Tremendousness, director. Science of Gratitude. YouTube, 6 Oct. 2016, https://youtu.be/JMd1CcGZYwU. Accessed 19 Aug. 2022.
Wildermuth, Erin. "The Science of Decision Fatigue." Full Focus, 11 Sept. 2018, https://fullfocus.co/the-science-of-decision-fatigue/.

www.ingramcontent.com/pod-product-compliance
Lightning Source LLC
Chambersburg PA
CBHW040202160726
48006CB00014B/1868